DIET FOR WEIGHT LOSS

Lose Weight and Keep it off. Starting now

JOHN OLUDIRAN

ISBN: 9798351335063

DEDICATION

I dedicate this book to the Almighty God for is Grace and Opportunity I received for writing this Script.

CONTENTS

INTRODUCTION

One of the issues that most People are likely worried with is weight loss. Numerous health problems and other challenges can be brought on by the widespread obesity epidemic. It's becoming more and more crucial to lose weight because eating only processed meals can be so unhealthy, not merely as a trend or aesthetic standard. In North America, processed foods are likely one of the main causes of obesity-related deaths.

Processed meals pose a huge number of risks. They include several carbohydrates and hidden fats, for instance. The foods are processed, and the ingredients are really unnatural. Numerous health issues, such as diabetes and hypertension, might be exacerbated by them. To avoid high fructose corn syrup when browsing the aisles of a grocery shop is probably next to impossible. High fructose corn syrup, which is often known as pure sugar, is extremely unhealthy. But you have a harder time eliminating this kind of sugar from your body.

When it comes to losing weight, everyone is searching for a magic solution. It can be quite simple to put on weight and very challenging to lose it once you do. If this is the case, returning to the state of being you desire to be in may seem nearly impossible. Our habits and behaviors have the power to mold and form our bodies, which can be thought of as instruments. Any diet won't work until you first change yourself and your perspective. Only then will you be able to maintain the consistency of effort necessary to genuinely lose weight and adhere to the recommended diet.

Whether or not you are fed every day, developing malnutrition is actually quite straightforward. The majority of the time when we eat, junk food is what keeps us alive and keeps us nourished. at least in the immediate future. However, because you are not eating things that are nourishing to your body, it will reduce your lifetime over time.

How then can you start to reduce weight and give yourself the nutrition you require to survive rather than just get by in life? By adhering to the Infallible diet's rules,

The Infallible diet will provide you with all the knowledge you need to start altering your life right now, even if your goal isn't merely weight loss but rather to improve your lifestyle.

1 Tracking Your Current Diet

When it comes to your weight reduction attempts, what you eat can make or break your efforts. If you're not willing to monitor your diet and identify where it needs to change, you may never achieve your weight loss potential or objectives.

Keeping track of the diet you are now following is one of the best strategies to start a reliable diet. What do you regularly eat? What is the fundamental structure of your diet? Do you give yourself way too much freedom when it comes to taking care of your body, or are you trying your best? Do you feel compelled to consume fast food constantly because you are busy and exhausted? Or, do you simply lack culinary skills and find yourself getting impatient with the amount of time and effort it can take to make a nutritious meal at the end of a long day?

Whatever the situation, keeping track of your nutrition is an excellent approach to start making changes in your life. But how do you start keeping track of your nutrition right now? You should, first and foremost, keep a journal or notebook in which you record your daily activities. Start at the beginning, and if you struggle to drink water instead of other sugary and unhealthy beverages, you should also include the water you have already consumed. Starting at that moment you get out of bed and keep going till you've had your fill for the day. If you get up to fetch a snack, either write these things down once they happen if you feel too exhausted, or save them for the next day. The best outcomes, however, come from being totally honest about your eating habits and from recording them right away.

It can take some time for the majority of people to form a habit. In fact, biologically it can be 7 days before a habit is formed by repeating positive behaviors. You'd be shocked at how difficult it is to recognize oneself after those new habits are ingrained. You might come to see that you are a powerful person who is capable of making significant changes for both yourself and your environment, as opposed to live your life consumed by the impact of your bad habits and patterns.

Anyone makes mistakes, and after engaging in a

negative habit for a while, it can be challenging to change. The secret, though, lies in accepting where you are at and being utterly honest and truthful about it, rather than in shaming yourself. It is something that may be incredibly healing and a very helpful tool in making great life changes, now and for the days to come. Not everyone is able to examine the hard truths of a situation with the courage it takes to implement changes utilizing the information they have observed about themselves.

2 Starting a Food Journal

It is a good idea to start a food journal once you have started tracking your current diet and have a solid understanding of what it is that you are doing that may prohibit you from moving forward with your weight loss journey. An excellent tool for keeping track of recipes you wish to make and developing meal plans that will help you stick to a healthy diet rich in fruits and vegetables is a food journal. Additionally, it will greatly assist you in developing the kind of accountability you require to make good adjustments and maintain them.

The same record you used to determine the overall composition of your daily diet might serve as the basis for your food journal. However, it is not necessary. To keep your meal journal, you could alternatively use a different notebook. The food journal is a highly helpful tool for maintaining a healthy diet and assisting with weight loss. It can be difficult to keep in mind that we are keeping on track for a reason if you don't have something that will assist you take responsibility for what you are putting into your body every day.

Humans are prone to short-term thinking and are

unable to make long-term plans. Planning for the future, such as keeping a food journal to help you keep track of the ingredients and meals you need or want to try, can really give you a solid foundation and a once-in-a-lifetime chance to see how every little decision you make can either improve your future or keep you from becoming the person you want to be.

It will be easier for you to consider your daily decisions more carefully if you are aware of the enormous effects of every decision you make. When you don't understand, it can be very difficult to stick to a plan or routine that gives your body the nourishment it needs for healing in order to grow.
Make sure that you are being honest with your entries in order to get the most out of a food journal. Attempt to note the meals you are consuming as soon as you eat them, and try to write in it every day. If you'd like, you could also keep track of their nutritional worth so you can keep track of what you're eating each day and won't be caught off guard at the end of the week if you discover you've gained or lost weight.

Next, as you may have thought given the word "journal" involved, you should also keep track of how you felt after consuming each food as well as how you felt before consuming each food. It's important to take into account how you felt after consuming these foods because, if you can precisely gauge your reactions, you can learn a lot about a food's nutritional value and compatibility with your body. For instance, if you discover you have a nut or soy intolerance but no overt allergy, you might discover that you feel angrier, moodier, or more agitated after consuming certain foods. This is due to the fact that your body has detected a threat and is sending you a stress signal to deal with the situation. Keep a close eye on what your body responds to and what probably doesn't. This will give you the ability to thoroughly and personally evaluate which foods are best for you. In this way, you will actually comprehend why some foods are bad for you while others may not be as challenging for you to love.

Overall, keeping a food journal can help you learn more about yourself and your eating habits. The majority of civilizations view eating as a communal, spiritual experience that should be savored. In North American for example, more thoughts is given to savoring out meals rather than being able to take solace in being aware of the precise interactions our bodies will have with foods once they are consumed and the therapeutic effects this brings.
Knowing our bodies and being in touch with

ourselves enough to make good decisions as frequently as possible is one of the most crucial elements in developing a diet plan that will work every time. It can be quite difficult to act in our own best interests when we are out of sync with ourselves. But keeping a food diary is a fantastic way to help us get our bodies in shape and minds together and concentrated on a crucial component of enhancing our health and wellbeing.

3 Getting Rid of Problem Foods

Everybody has their vices, and these problematic meals can lead even the most well-intentioned dieters astray. If we're not careful, it might be very difficult for her to retain her composure. This is particularly true of eating habits since, most of the time, we form them in an effort to find a quick cure for raging hunger. When we can't quickly solve the problem, we become upset and frustrated, and frequently give up on cooking altogether. Have you ever had one of those days where you could prepare something simple at home but instead chose to go shopping for something simple?

The moment has come to start recognizing these behaviors and examining how they are impacting you over time. Sometimes, relying too heavily on quick and simple foods might be really risky. Even if it seems like a quick fix and you feel good because of all the fats and sugars giving your body chemical reactions that convince you that you are enjoying this food and that is what your body wants or needs, processed foods come with a whole host of potential health problems that can make your body suffer over time.

Every home has issue foods, and they could be

hiding in every cabinet or cupboard, just waiting to be found. The first indication that you should get rid of problem foods that you have at home is if you discover that you have to resist the impulse to eat them.
First and foremost, you should stop drinking sodas and other sugary beverages. The majority of people are unaware of how much sugar is in juice. We believe it to be healthy because it is made of fruit, yet fruit is loaded with natural sugars, and when it is juiced, we lose the fruit's beneficial natural fibers. Instead, we typically consume a mixture of naturally occurring added sugars as well as concentrated fruit juice sugars that are present in the juice. This also applies to other supposedly healthy meals like yogurt and granola bars. They contain a lot of sugar, making it nearly impossible to avoid them when consumed and check for outcomes.

You could definitely completely cut out sugar if you wanted to, and the results would come quite quickly as well. Generally speaking, make an effort to keep your daily sugar intake to no more than 30 g. This can be challenging since, when you start to read the ingredient lists on your foods and soft drinks, you discover that the majority of these beverages include two servings, although the recommended maximum amount of sugar to consume for weight reduction is one serving.

Attempt not to feel guilty about throwing away food that will result in future health issues or weight gain. At times, this is the only option to bring about significant change. The only way to start getting stronger than our destructive desires is to try.

Instead, evaluate the unhealthy foods that are a frequent part of your diet and actively work to eliminate them. You will be on the right road in avoiding these meals if you either get rid of the ones you already own or refrain from purchasing them in the first place.

The following are some examples of foods you may want to avoid:

Processed foods, candies, sugary foods, fatty foods, salty meals, sugary foods, soft drinks, and juices are all examples of processed foods.

- Smoothies with a fruit ratio of greater than two parts three portions vegetables
- White flour products and starchy foods like potatoes (pasta noodles, etc.)

Make every effort to avoid the foods you know will be harmful and will impede your efforts to lose weight by using your common sense and taking sensible precautions.

Most people have an innate sense of what meals are unhealthy for us when they see them. Making the most of the foods we know are healthy for us while avoiding the quick and simple ones is typically a test of willpower. Your nutritious meals might become quick and simple for you if you pre-prepare them. It all depends on your point of view. Getting rid of troublesome meals shouldn't be a difficulty for you at all if you retrain your brain to think that you are choosing what is best for yourself.

4 Slow and Steady Wins the Race

Starting a new, healthy habit might be more difficult than most people believe, but if you are committed to reaching your objectives, nothing should stand in your way. But a lot of what keeps us from achieving our goals is a mental block that may cause a lot of interruptions and disturbances in our life. Fortunately for us, there are steps we can take to start taking care of our bodies and brains as well as psychologically preparing for the demanding task ahead of us.

Realistic expectations are a terrific method to help us get ahead before we even start. Don't count on having a healthy meal just one day a week to help you lose weight. That is actually very far from the truth. You must make sure that you are doing everything in your ability to stick with your goals, even when you relapse, if you want to lose weight.

When we are not being realistic, reaching our goals becomes more difficult. We need to take things slowly while trying to create a new habit. Instead of setting unreasonable goals for yourself that will be practically hard to achieve and sustain, introduce it

gradually, in little amounts, and over time. Do your best to adopt tiny adjustments gradually until they feel like a natural part of your life, rather than making multiple big lifestyle changes all at once.
We must begin modestly. Overextending ourselves is the surest path to failure. We should be cautious while introducing new habits into our life. Start out by taking baby steps. For instance, try beginning by eliminating one harmful habit at a time rather than putting out every unhealthy food to which you are attracted. Before eliminating another food that you know you should stop eating, wait about a week after you've taken out the first one.

Although it may seem tedious, this approach is a surefire way to ensure that the improvements you are trying to make stick. It is incredibly important to be able to take a step back and give your body the time to become used to making better choices instead of overtaxing your head with a lot of different stressful changes.

Try to be gentle with yourself when making dietary adjustments because it can be physically taxing. Relapses can and probably will happen, but you must keep in mind that you are doing this to improve your health, not to punish yourself. It's okay if you make a mistake. But try to keep moving forward and leave your mistakes in the past. Avoid letting a single error lead you back to your unhealthy way of life. Although it could seem challenging at first, you'll be amazed by how simple it is to start adapting to the lifestyle of making healthy, body-aware decisions that will benefit you and open the door to a healthier future for yourself.

Don't go overboard. You must be certain that you are tackling your issues in a way that will provide you the tools you require to succeed. When you are unable to do so, things become challenging. In order to start forming all the new habits you want to adopt to make your lifestyle as healthy as it can be, you can try setting aside a date every two weeks to start introducing new habits and eating modifications.

And this doesn't apply to only altering your diet and eliminating bad foods from your way of life. This applies to pretty much every lifestyle decision you might make. For instance, if you wanted to start learning a new language, you could start out slowly by establishing a new routine that involved studying that language once a week. You may gradually increase the frequency of your language practice to two to three times per week, or even daily, if you set aside time for it. You will eventually be able to form a habit that will get you closer and closer to the life you have always imagined for yourself, as long as you start off slowly.

You can definitely succeed in achieving your objectives. You only need to approach them with realistic expectations of yourself and the biological truth that some habits can occasionally come more effortlessly while others take a long time to form. In either case, avoid trying to make a lot of adjustments at once in order to avoid taxing your brain. You'll have the framework you need to make long-lasting decisions that will improve your life moving forward if you can gradually adapt to the changes.

5 Combining Exercise for Best Results

In conclusion, you want to burn more calories than you take in. To do this, you need to create a regimen that combines both healthy eating and activities that will help you lose weight while simultaneously feeding your body, muscles, and mind.

It might be challenging to burn calories, particularly if your lifestyle is unchanging. It might be challenging to move your body and engage in the exercise you need to perform each day to maintain your blood flowing normally if you spend the entire day sat in front of a computer. Due to this, it is even more difficult to maintain a healthy weight and burn calories, let alone get rid of extra body fat that has accumulated.

Living a sedentary lifestyle is extremely harmful to our bodies. Without taking into account what we need to do physically to support a sure-fire and surefire strategy of losing weight, we can't just go on a diet and expect fast and healthy weight loss outcomes. It's acceptable if you don't want to lose weight. To ensure that you are not hurting yourself, it is still crucial to keep up a regular workout schedule. Lack of activity makes it challenging for the body to get rid of toxins, particularly those that are accumulated inside our body fat. This may make losing weight all but difficult. It is challenging for us to get rid of the extra body fat inside of us since toxins frequently bind to our fat cells.

Because of this, exercise is crucial. We can start to gain muscle while also starting to sweat away the toxins and other harmful substances from our systems. Building muscle enables us to burn fat continuously throughout the day. Strength training is actually a terrific strategy to develop the muscles we need to keep a healthy metabolism and be able to flourish. Muscles enable the body to continuously burn the fuel we consume when we are creating them. We start to shed fat and truly start to see results in our weight reduction efforts when we are using up more calories than we are consuming.

The addition of aerobic exercises might be quite helpful as well. If you are not exercising and keeping your heart rate up, it is difficult for your body to shed weight. Cardio exercise increases the deficit between calories ingested and calories burned by burning a lot of calories. This indicates that you will lose weight. This is especially true if you choose healthy foods throughout the day rather than unwise foods that make you gain weight or cause you to hold on to stubborn fat instead of burning it through exercise and wise eating.

Without exercise, you might be able to lose weight, but the results will be minor at best. Moving your body and getting your blood flowing will unquestionably help you lose weight and get started on the path to having the figure you've always desired when you follow a dependable diet plan. Because you deserve to be the best version of yourself, and exercising will enable you to do that.

6 Creating a Calorie Deficit for Weight Loss

The majority of people detest the thought of calculating calories, and they should. It can lead to an unhealthy focus on your body image and the foods you are willing to eat, and it is dull, awful, and uninteresting. It can be a very constrained way to live. However, if you stick to the weight loss diet plan and consume a diet high in vegetables and protein while combining it with muscle-building exercises that enable you to burn through your fat in no time at all, you'll discover that creating a calorie deficit really isn't all that difficult and it doesn't have to be very restrictive in the foods that you eat at all!

As long as you are consuming foods that are strengthening your body rather than making it harder for you to sustain yourself and maintain a healthy lifestyle, creating a calorie deficit using the healthy food choices advised in this book should be simple. It is an excellent method for ensuring that your diet will be beneficial to you rather than detrimental.

The average amount of calories in one pound of fat

is 3,500. You must be able to burn around that many calories every day, excluding what you eat, in order to lose one pound of fat. To lose a pound of fat each week at this point, it would typically make a difference to reduce calories by roughly 500 per day.

A daily calorie deficit of 500 calories or fewer is considered to be reasonably healthy. In light of what you generally eat, you must either reduce the number of calories you consume at meals or engage in physical activity to generate a calorie deficit. Of course, as was already indicated, the quickest way to guarantee weight loss is to combine a balanced diet with exercise.

Most of us are aware of the fact that no diet is perfect. In actuality, a lot of fad diets are quite dangerous and hazardous. Some of these might even have long-term health effects. Long-term damage to your body might result from various diets, including the hcg diet and others that may encourage dangerous behaviors or the use of unproven medications. Consider all the benefits that will come with losing weight, rather than letting the promise of quick weight loss deceive you. Losing weight will be the least of your concerns if you have sagging skin and a host of other health issues. Does it sound like it would be worthwhile? Because it isn't, that is.

The key to losing weight is to generate a calorie deficit, which you will do if you consistently track your calories, make an effort to eat nutritional meals, and combine a healthy diet with consistent exercise. You might find it helpful to meet with a nutritionist so they can advise you on how to take your unique needs into account as you embark on this new adventure in your life. By doing it this manner, you may complete every task quickly and carefully while also treating your body with the respect it merits.

7 Introducing Fruits and Vegetables for Weight Loss

Healthy and natural foods are one thing that is severely lacking in the normal ordinary People diet. Fruits and vegetables are frequently overlooked in favor of convenient canned items, which are typically stretched-out replicas of their previous nutritionally dense selves. Dependence on canned and processed meals can be quite harmful. If you're not careful, they can quickly make you gain weight and deprive your body of nutrients because they are packed with hidden carbohydrates and fats.

Many people who are obsessed with reducing weight don't seem to comprehend the importance of fruits and vegetables in this regard. In addition to preventing hunger, they are high in fiber and water, which aid in digestion and help your body get rid of extra waste. Additionally, you might discover that you feel fuller more quickly as a result of those fibers. Additionally, there isn't really a limit on how many servings of fruits and vegetables you should have each day. If you are not diabetic or have another ailment that could need you to avoid natural sugars, they make excellent snacks for hungry dieters.

The metabolism can be boosted by eating fruits and vegetables, which can provide a satisfying snack that is low in calories, high in fiber, and high in water content. This indicates that you normally don't need to worry too much about putting on weight if you eat as many vegetables as you like. This is actually wonderful news since you can consume a ton of nutritious meals that will provide you a ton of sustenance instead of starving yourself. Your ability to engage in the other fantastic components of weight loss, such as being active and having a regular exercise regimen, will be aided by healthy eating.

Additionally, it will keep your mind sharp, which is beneficial if you want to start a change in lifestyle like this. It will be extremely unlikely that you will want to make the necessary changes if you are feeling exhausted, lethargic, and miserable. It will also be very challenging for the changes you do make to stick once you start to make an effort. However, a terrific approach to start a path that will bring you healing and enhance your health is by consuming foods that are nutritious for you, help you maintain your energy levels, and help you stay focused.

In fact, food is revered as medicine in many civilizations. It is thought that eating correctly and at the right times of the day would enable you to keep a healthier body as well as a better mood and spirit overall. Due to the fact that so many of the foods used as medicine really have anti-inflammatory and antibacterial characteristics, including them regularly in your diet will help you stay healthy. The ancient healing art of Ayurveda has been around for millennia and is still in use today. That is supported by some science, in fact. You will be able to give your immune system the resources it requires to fight off illness and disease if you eat healthfully.

Even though it is well known that fresh fruits and vegetables are bursting with the vitamins and minerals our bodies require to thrive, they are sadly too frequently absent from the typical People diet. It might be challenging to keep up high energy levels if the right food types aren't included in our meals. At least, you can start to feel a difference in your mood when you are eating a normal amount of fruits and vegetables.

Additionally, you'll start to notice a change in your weight. Your body will start to eliminate the toxins that tie fat to them if you go from a diet high in starchy and carb-filled foods to one higher in water-based foods that are full of fiber. This will enable you to start losing weight more quickly.

8 The Importance of Drinking Water for Weight Loss

In the beginning, most people put on a lot of weight due to how challenging it is to refrain from drinking sugar-laden beverages. Smoothies, soda, and juice—all of which have higher than recommended sugar levels—make up a large portion of many people's daily meals. If this problem isn't resolved, your body may find it difficult to process the extra sugars you are ingesting and may easily start to put on weight. It is harmful for the body to be so continuously overburdened with sugars.

Most people don't realize how important drinking water is for losing weight. In truth, people don't give water nearly enough credit, especially in western cultures where the general public prefers sugary and caffeinated drinks over water. No matter how much time and effort you put into it, these drinks are calorie-dense and might make it seem hard to start losing weight. Water is a low-calorie substitute that benefits in a wide range of other ways in addition to aiding in weight loss.

Water is hydrating and moisturizing, and it can help us overcome skin issues and give our skin a radiant glow. Additionally, it can help to produce skin that is touchably soft and well-hydrated. It can also aid in the reduction of headaches and the elimination of toxins from the body when we are able to give our bodies the right amount of water.

Actually, it may happen rather frequently for our bodies to mix up hunger and thirst signals. It is advised that you start drinking water before eating if you feel your stomach grumbling. You can start to tell the difference between hunger and thirst. It can also assist you in avoiding overeating because you mistook your body's response to thirst for hunger. When your stomach grumbles or you feel hungry, try to drink some water right away because thirst and hunger both signal a need for food. Many people misunderstand this, but it doesn't imply that you should eat whenever you feel hungry. Just use this as a general guideline, and you might be amazed at how simple it is to avoid consuming extra calories.

Water can inhibit hunger, which is a fact that not many people are aware of. In other words, if you choose to drink enough water, you will eventually notice that you are less hungry during the day. This can be particularly true if you have a glass of water before eating. In order to avoid overeating at meals, it will help you control and suppress your appetite.

If you struggle with portion control, this approach will be extremely helpful. One of the healthiest and most organic ways to stop yourself from overeating is to drink a glass of water before a meal. Getting enough water can also help your body function properly and enable you to concentrate. Similar to eating enough fruits and vegetables, the human body tends to get lethargic and unpleasant when not obtaining enough water in the diet. We are built to function optimally in environments with plenty of water. It is comparable to the fuel that keeps our bodies functioning at their peak.

Typically, 64 ounces of water each day are needed to keep things running smoothly. You will be able to control your appetite better and concentrate more clearly as a result. Being mentally strong will help you maintain a strong physical state as well. In order to achieve your goals, you will need to be extremely focused and persistent. If you are taking care of your body's fundamental needs, this will be much easier for you to do.

The idea that drinking water can help you increase your metabolism just by doing so may be the most amazing thing about it. It prepares your body to burn calories for a longer period of time and enables the body to burn fat for energy.

Overall, using water as a means of losing weight is a terrific method to effortlessly support a failsafe diet. This is another important reason why water helps with weight reduction. It will be especially effective if you stop drinking other beverages, notably soda and other high-sugar juices and similar things. The easiest method to lose weight is to attempt to limit your consumption of sugar, and switching to water from sugary beverages is a wonderful way to start burning the calories you already have in your body rather than consuming more.

Try tea or infuse your water with fruits or veggies if you find that drinking water and nothing else isn't working for you (perhaps because it is too plain). If you like the taste of cucumber, specifically, cucumber is a really delightful method to infuse water and urge you to drink more. If not, you have a number of other good choices, such as but not restricted to watermelon, lemon, or strawberries.

These are all wonderful and delectable methods to increase your water intake without significantly raising the caloric content of your water as you would if you drank soda or juice.

Especially if you have seen all the documentaries and other study regarding juicing, you might be thinking if it is a smart idea to juice. The plain truth is that store-bought juices include significant amounts of sugar from the fruits they contain as well as extra sugars added during the production process. It is not wholesome. Juicing fruits and vegetables, on the other hand, is a very different matter.

The problem with this is that using a juicer to consume your fruits and veggies instead of eating them would remove the healthy fibers that make fruits and vegetables so good for the body from the beverage. For maximum outcomes, make sure to include the fibers, at least a few, to juice rather than drinking pulp-free juice. Additionally, you should refrain from juicing a large number of fruits at once because you will effectively be ingesting sugar water. Fruits are a rich source of natural sugar, thus consuming too much juice made largely of fruit might be harmful.

In order to gain the additional benefits of the fibers that make fruits and vegetables particularly healthy and helpful for weight reduction, the idea is to drink juices that are two parts vegetable and one part fruit and add some pulp. Juicing will be covered in more detail in the last chapter since it offers a number of weight loss suggestions and techniques. particularly if you are considering a wide range of food options.

Drinking plenty of water is typically the best thing you can do to increase your metabolism and kick start your weight loss. Without an opportunity to eliminate toxins from the body and revitalize the cells, our bodies store both water and fat, which can make it very difficult to get the bodies we want. Reaching your objectives might be simpler than you think. To make your diet as risk-free as it can be, just make sure you are consuming about 64 ounces of water each day so that you can fully benefit from water intake. You'll be happy that you did. It is such a straightforward and practical tool for assisting with both weight loss and enhancing our general health.

9 LEAN MEATS AND HEALTHY PROTEIN SOURCES

Protein is excellent for the body for a number of reasons, as has been repeatedly demonstrated. In addition to helping you gain muscle mass, it also tends to help ward off hunger, which can be a fantastic way to enforce portion control when it seems to be the most difficult.

Nevertheless, certain protein sources are better than others, and if you want to ensure that your body is healing as soon as possible while growing muscle that helps to burn fat quickly, you want to avoid protein sources that will actually be adding more fat to your body.

The greatest sources of protein for you are those that are lean, particularly if you want to lose weight successfully and go to any lengths to sustain the lifestyle that you are forging for yourself. These protein sources are crucial to your weight loss efforts, and the next paragraph lists the greatest plant- and animal-based sources of lean protein that you can locate.

One of the best sources of lean protein is eggs. They contain a lot of this particular nutrient and are satisfying. And you don't need to consume a lot of them to receive a lot of protein and a strong energy boost. This is a great snack to have post work out to help you to build muscle and burn fat all day long!

Lean meats are mostly poultry based, such as the white meat found in turkey or chicken. Red meats are more fatty and less lean, which can have an adverse effect on weight loss. Other lean protein sources include soy and seafood, though be careful about where you get your seafood from.

Due to the coal factories being so close to the coastlines, some seafood is unfortunately tainted with contaminants like mercury. You should also be aware of farmed fish. If you're interested in including seafood in your diet, research ethically grown seafood. Also, keep in mind that the quickest path to sustaining a healthy diet for the rest of your life is to make wise and informed food decisions.

Nuts and seeds, such as sunflower seeds, almonds, pistachios, cashews, walnuts, pumpkin seeds, and other well-known seed and nut kinds that are rich with proteins and good fats, are also excellent sources of lean protein.

Healthy fats are crucial for weight loss as well. You will inevitably gain weight if you eat bad fats. Healthy fats, on the other hand, are crucial to the body's structure and should be included in the diet.

They support your body and give you a fantastic source of energy without making losing weight too challenging.

Nut butters and seeds, as well as foods like avocados and olives, are examples of healthy fats. Even olive oil is a wonderful source of healthy fat and has long-term benefits for the body as opposed to short-term drawbacks. If you can find a good source of seafood, eating fish is a terrific method to maintain the body slim and healthy without giving up the rich and tasty meals that fill your body and mind with satisfaction. Fish is another source of healthy fat.

The distinction between lean and fatty meat is frequently the cause. Since all meat has some fat, eating fish and other lean seafood is extremely beneficial to your health. These are stuffed with good fat, not unhealthy fat. Because the animals from which red meat originates are larger, stockier, and have a different type of diet than livestock that produces lean meat sources for consumption, red meat in particular is higher in fat. Fish is undoubtedly the finest option for anyone who will be consuming meat for a prolonged period of time in order to sustain themselves and try to live as healthily as possible because it does not include saturated fats like the other varieties of meat.

There are advantages and disadvantages to eating

meat overall, and if you are a vegan or vegetarian or just don't consume a lot of meat, there are different protein options you can choose from. Keep in mind that both tempeh and tofu are made of soy, and that there are other foods like nuts, nut butters, seeds, and even some leafy green vegetables that can give you a healthy amount of protein as well.

The most important factor in developing a healthy lifestyle that will provide you a surefire strategy to lose weight and keep it off, starting right now, is educating yourself and starting out slowly.

10 Planning Meals and Other Tips and Tricks.

Any lifestyle change will require planning before you start. It will fail if you aren't totally prepared for it. The mental and emotional difficulties that come with weight loss and the changes that must be made both mentally and physically before we can lose weight and keep it off are generally not covered in diet plans.

Before you can ever solve your sadness, you must be able to identify its underlying cause. Why, for instance, are you a chronic overeater? What emotional hole are you attempting to fill? If yes, what caused it to be there and how can it be fixed? Are you only having trouble exercising self-control? If so, why do you believe that might be the case and what can you do to strengthen your reliability? Or is your problem more a result of the fact that you don't have a lot of cooking experience and tend to rely on the simplest dishes? Do you feel pressed for time and that cooking requires more time than it is worth? If so, research simple meal preparation manuals and advice that will assist you in preparing meals at home in a style that you are comfortable with and that will sustain you.

If you eat meat, reading about the Paleo diet is a

terrific place to start. The paleo diet aims to nourish your body as naturally as possible while avoiding manufactured meals and the high levels of sugar they contain, which make weight loss challenging.

Juicing can be beneficial, particularly if you struggle to consume fruits and vegetables in their natural states. Adding apples to juices is a terrific approach to get yourself interested in them. Apples are healthy and naturally delicious but not overpowering. An apple or two won't hurt anything as long as you are reintroducing some of the natural fibers from the fruits and veggies to your drink. In reality, whether or not the juice contains vegetables you may not like, it is a fantastic method to add nutrients and a lovely, sweet flavor!

You should disregard the following advice if you don't mind drinking water and don't think juicing would be a necessary technique to include a diversity of drinks in your diet. The majority of people I know struggle to consume the recommended quantity of water each day and instead choose more palatable beverages. Water may be made a little more interesting by adding diversity, and flavoring it with fruits and vegetables is a great way to do so.

Another tip is to wait until you have consumed at least half of your recommended daily amount of water before indulging in other beverages that you believe to be somewhat healthy but more flavored or sweet. After drinking the recommended amount of water each day, you can treat yourself to something else that could be a little sweeter.

Although it is recommended to avoid all sugary and processed drinks in general in order to have the greatest effects, it is more important that you are living your life in a way that is bearable and manageable for you and you are making conscious choices in what you consume.

The 'diet for weight loss' true goal is to help you develop the resolve to make good decisions that will alter how you perceive food. Don't worry if you believe that your options are limited because you lack culinary creativity when preparing nutritious cuisine. Every new experience in the kitchen should be viewed as an opportunity to learn more, so take this as a chance to do so. There are things that can make it easier, even if things get off to a rocky start. For instance, planning your meals in advance is a terrific method to help you start going. You can learn how to plan your meals throughout the week by using one of the many meal planners available online. Follow the diet recommended in this book. fruits, vegetables, lean proteins, and meats. Consume starches sparingly, no more than once or twice each week as a mainstay. They are full of sugars that make you feel even more hungry, causing you to eat more food that ultimately turns into fat in your body. It will undoubtedly be challenging at first. Drink at least 64 ounces of water each day and stay away from processed foods and sugar the dreaded plague.

the paleo diet is a fantastic overall guideline to follow; staying away from the bad foods can really help you keep balanced, provide you a reliable approach to diet, and help you adjust your lifestyle in a way that works best for you. one that is certain to endure.

CONCLUSION

Nowadays, everyone is searching for the finest diet to follow in order to lose weight and keep it off. a quick, simple fix for the issues that have started to afflict us as a result of our prolonged acceptance of an unhealthy way of life. Most people, however, overlook the truth that the biggest benefit is actually produced by our own thinking and habits. We rely on other people to make an effort to assist us in trying to dig ourselves out of a hole that only we have the means to escape. Your life is in your hands. You will be in charge of making the decisions necessary to alter your way of life. You are more, too than capable of accomplishing it.

Start off modestly. Take it slow. Divide up your goals into digestible bits, and then confidently start pursuing them. You must possess the strength and confidence to get back up even if you relapse or fall. Success is entirely up to you, and the diet for weight loss will only be that way if you make it work for you rather than the other way around.

Many people don't seem to realize how significant you are, though. You are worthwhile. Because we don't always value ourselves and lack the self-love and self-discipline required to create the life of our choosing, we punish ourselves and make poor decisions. But starting right now, all of that can change. You will have the tools at your disposal to make the changes you need to make if you are prepared to look at yourself honestly and how you got to where you are now.

What would really make a difference is to simplify things rather than adding more and more fad diets and fads to your life. Choose straightforward foods. Consume wholesome, nutritious foods that are low in fat and sugar. Avoid eating foods that you are already aware are bad for you. These straightforward rules of thumb will become increasingly difficult to follow unless all the underlying causes of your difficulty with healthy eating are resolved.

You are where the failsafe diet starts and stops. No matter how many diet books and pieces of advice you read, in the end, it is up to you to decide how to live your life. You will have the resources you need to succeed and start living the life you deserve, starting right now, if you follow the advice in the "Diet for weight loss" book.

www.ingramcontent.com/pod-product-compliance
Lightning Source LLC
LaVergne TN
LVHW020524160826
845677LV00015B/3880

* 9 7 9 8 3 5 1 3 3 5 0 6 3 *